MARC REXUS

Rising Above: A Journey of Pregnancy and Healthcare for the Black Woman

Disclaimer:

While the advice and information in this book are believed to be accurate and based on reliable sources, they are not intended to replace consultation with a qualified healthcare professional. Every pregnancy and individual's health circumstances are unique. Therefore, any readers of this book are strongly encouraged to consult with their own healthcare provider before making any decisions about their health or treatment during pregnancy. No information in this book should be used to disregard, delay, or refuse treatment by a licensed healthcare provider. The author and publisher expressly disclaim responsibility for any adverse effects that may result from the use or application of the information contained in this book.

First edition

This book was professionally typeset on Reedsy.
Find out more at reedsy.com

Contents

1

Chapter 1: The Reality of Black Maternal Health

E very woman embarking on the journey of motherhood deserves comprehensive, compassionate healthcare that ensures her safety and that of her baby. Yet, the American healthcare system continues to grapple with severe racial and ethnic disparities, particularly in maternal health. Alarmingly, Black women have consistently experienced higher maternal mortality rates and pregnancy-related complications than their White counterparts. This chapter aims to shed light on the harsh realities of Black maternal health, explore the root causes of these disparities, and underscore the urgency for systemic changes.

The Stark Statistics

In the United States, Black women are three to four times more likely to die from pregnancy-related complications than White women, according to data from the Centers for Disease Control and Prevention (CDC). This disparity persists across all income and education levels. Further, Black women also face a higher risk of severe morbidity, which refers to unexpected outcomes of labor and delivery that result in significant short- or long-term consequences to a woman's health.

The Underlying Causes

Several interrelated factors contribute to these disparities, ranging from systemic and social determinants to biological factors.

1. **Racism and Bias in Healthcare:** Black women often encounter both overt and subtle racial bias within the healthcare system. They are less likely to have their pain and symptoms taken seriously, leading to delays in diagnosis and treatment. This unconscious bias among medical professionals can lead to inadequate care and adverse health outcomes.
2. **Socioeconomic Factors:** Although these disparities persist across all income levels, socioeconomic factors play a significant role. Black women are more likely to lack access to quality prenatal care, face financial barriers to healthcare, and live in medically underserved areas.
3. **Chronic Stress and Weathering:** The term "weathering" describes the way in which chronic exposure to social, economic, and political inequities leads to deteriorating physical health. For Black women, the constant stress of systemic racism can lead to pre-existing conditions that complicate pregnancy and childbirth.

An Urgent Call to Action

The maternal health crisis among Black women is a public health emergency that demands immediate action. Addressing this crisis requires a multi-faceted approach, including healthcare policy reform, improved access to prenatal and postnatal care, and comprehensive bias training for healthcare professionals.

Moreover, it is crucial to empower Black women with knowledge and resources to navigate the healthcare system effectively. This includes teaching them about potential pregnancy complications, their rights as patients, and the importance of self-advocacy.

In the following chapters, we will explore practical steps and strategies for Black women to overcome these challenges and ensure the best possible health outcomes for themselves and their babies. The journey ahead is daunting, but change is not only possible—it is imperative.

2

Chapter 2: Understanding the Healthcare System

The American healthcare system is notoriously complex, with its intricate interplay of public and private entities, insurers, providers, and consumers. For pregnant Black women, comprehending this system becomes particularly crucial to ensuring their well-being and that of their unborn child. This chapter aims to offer a basic understanding of the healthcare system's structure, the intricacies of insurance, and the ways these elements affect the maternal health journey.

The Structure of the Healthcare System

The U.S. healthcare system is a mix of public and private sectors. The public sector includes programs like Medicaid and Medicare, administered by the government and often serving low-income individuals, the elderly, and the disabled. The private sector comprises private health insurance companies, usually provided through employers.

Healthcare Providers: These are the professionals or organizations that provide health services. This includes doctors, nurses, midwives, hospitals, clinics, and other medical facilities.

Health Insurance Companies: These are entities that offer insurance policies covering a range of healthcare services. These companies often have agreements with certain healthcare providers forming 'networks.'

Navigating Insurance

Understanding insurance jargon and policies is a critical step in effectively accessing and utilizing healthcare services.

Premiums: This is the amount you pay regularly (monthly, quarterly, annually) to maintain your insurance coverage.

Deductibles: This is the amount you must pay out-of-pocket for care before your insurance company starts to cover costs.

Co-pays and Co-insurance: These are your share of the costs of a healthcare service, paid out-of-pocket. Co-pay is a fixed amount, while co-insurance is a percentage of the total cost.

Out-of-pocket Maximum: The most you'll have to pay for covered services in a policy period. After you reach this amount, your health insurance will pay 100% of the costs of covered benefits.

In-network and Out-of-network: In-network providers have a contract with your insurance company to provide services at a discounted rate. Out-of-network providers don't have such a contract, and you may have to pay more to see them.

How Healthcare System Affects Your Maternal Health Journey

Navigating the healthcare system effectively can significantly impact your maternal health journey. Here are some key points to consider:

1. **Choice of Providers:** The choice of healthcare provider is crucial. Providers should not only be 'in-network' but also culturally competent and experienced in managing the unique health risks faced by Black women.

2. **Insurance Coverage:** Understanding what your insurance policy covers, from prenatal visits to childbirth to postpartum care, helps avoid unexpected expenses. It's also crucial to understand which tests, screenings, and procedures are covered.

3. **Medicaid and Pregnancy:** If you are eligible for Medicaid, be aware that it covers pregnancy and childbirth-related costs. Some states have expanded Medicaid coverage to low-income adults more broadly. If you're pregnant and uninsured, check your state's Medicaid rules.

The complexities of the healthcare system should not be a barrier to receiving quality care. Equip yourself with knowledge, ask questions, clarify doubts, and make informed decisions about your health and your baby's well-being. The subsequent chapters will further guide you on selecting a healthcare provider, understanding unique health risks, and advocating for yourself in the healthcare journey.

3

Chapter 3: Choosing the Right Healthcare Provider

The choice of a healthcare provider is a significant decision during pregnancy. The right provider understands and respects your cultural and personal needs, builds a relationship of trust, and plays a pivotal role in your pregnancy and childbirth journey. This chapter provides guidance on selecting a healthcare provider who can offer the best care for you and your baby.

Types of Maternity Healthcare Providers

There are several types of healthcare providers who can assist you during your pregnancy. The choice depends on your health, your pregnancy's risk level, and your personal preferences.

1. **Obstetrician-Gynecologists (OB-GYNs):** These are doctors specialized in women's health, including prenatal care, childbirth, and postpartum care.
2. **Family Physicians:** Some family physicians provide comprehensive healthcare, including prenatal and postnatal care.
3. **Midwives:** Certified nurse-midwives (CNMs) and certified professional midwives (CPMs) are trained to provide prenatal care and deliver babies, usually in lower-risk pregnancies.

4. **Maternal-Fetal Medicine (MFM) Specialists:** These are OB-GYNs with additional training in high-risk pregnancies.

Choosing a Culturally Competent Provider

Culturally competent healthcare providers understand and respect patients' cultural backgrounds, beliefs, and values. For Black women, choosing a provider who understands the unique challenges they face can significantly improve their healthcare experience.

1. **Ask for Recommendations:** Seek referrals from friends, family, or community groups. Hearing about others' experiences can provide insights into a provider's cultural competence.
2. **Research and Reviews:** Online platforms often have reviews from past patients. Look for reviews from patients who share your background and concerns.
3. **Direct Communication:** During your initial visit, have an open conversation about your expectations, fears, and needs. A competent provider will listen attentively, acknowledge your concerns, and provide clear and respectful responses.

Key Questions to Ask

It's crucial to ask potential providers questions about their experience, approach to care, and policies. Here are some key questions:

1. What is your experience with managing the unique health risks for Black women during pregnancy?
2. Can you provide information on your C-section rates?
3. How do you handle concerns about bias or discrimination in your practice?
4. What is your approach to pain management during labor?
5. Can I meet other members of your team who might be involved in my care?
6. What is your availability for questions or concerns outside of scheduled

appointments?

Red Flags to Watch Out For

It's important to trust your instincts and be aware of potential red flags:

1. Dismissive Behavior: A provider who dismisses your concerns or downplays your symptoms can jeopardize your health.
2. Poor Communication: If a provider consistently fails to explain things clearly or doesn't listen attentively, it can lead to misunderstandings and mistrust.
3. Lack of Respect for Your Cultural Values: If you feel a provider does not respect or acknowledge your cultural values and beliefs, they may not be the best fit for you.

Remember, your voice matters, and you have a right to quality, respectful care. Don't hesitate to switch providers if you feel uncomfortable or unheard. Your health and your baby's health are worth it.

4

Chapter 4: The Importance of Prenatal Care

P renatal care plays a vital role in the health of both the mother and the baby. Regular prenatal visits allow for early detection and management of potential health issues, ensuring the best possible outcomes for your pregnancy. This chapter delves into the importance of prenatal care, outlines the typical schedule of visits, and provides an overview of what to expect at each visit.

Why Prenatal Care Matters

Consistent prenatal care significantly contributes to a healthy pregnancy and birth. Here's why it's so important:

1. **Early Detection of Complications:** Regular check-ups allow healthcare providers to spot potential health problems early and take appropriate action. This is particularly important for Black women, who face higher risks of certain complications like preeclampsia and gestational diabetes.
2. **Education and Counseling:** Prenatal visits provide an opportunity to learn about the changes happening in your body, understand what to expect during each stage of pregnancy, and discuss any concerns or questions you have.
3. **Health Promotion:** Providers can offer guidance on maintaining a healthy lifestyle during pregnancy, including proper nutrition, safe physical activity, and the importance of mental health.

Typical Schedule of Prenatal Visits

The American College of Obstetricians and Gynecologists (ACOG) recommends the following schedule for low-risk pregnancies:

- Weekly visits until 28 weeks
- Every two weeks from 28 weeks to 36 weeks
- Weekly from 36 weeks to birth

High-risk pregnancies may require more frequent visits.

What to Expect at Each Visit

While the specifics of each visit can vary, here's a general idea of what to expect:

1. **Initial Visit (around 8 weeks):** This comprehensive visit may include a physical exam, Pap smear, blood and urine tests, and possibly an ultrasound. You'll discuss your health history, medications, lifestyle, and mental health.
2. **First Trimester:** Expect routine check-ups to monitor your blood pressure, weight, and baby's growth. You may also have screenings for genetic disorders.
3. **Second Trimester:** Along with routine check-ups, you'll have an anatomy ultrasound around 20 weeks to examine your baby's development. Screenings for gestational diabetes usually occur between 24-28 weeks.
4. **Third Trimester:** In addition to monitoring your and baby's health, visits may include checks for Group B strep, discussions about labor signs, and creating a birth plan.

Each visit is an opportunity to discuss any concerns or questions, including those about labor and delivery, breastfeeding, and newborn care.

A Note on Insurance Coverage

Most insurance plans, including Medicaid, cover prenatal care. If you're uninsured, explore options like Medicaid, the Children's Health Insurance

Program (CHIP), or local health department resources.

Prenatal care is a critical component of a healthy pregnancy. Ensure to attend all scheduled visits, advocate for yourself, ask questions, and follow through with recommended tests and screenings. Your active involvement can make a significant difference in your and your baby's health.

5

Chapter 5: Nutrition and Pregnancy

Proper nutrition during pregnancy is essential to support the healthy growth of your baby and maintain your well-being. However, it's important to remember that "eating for two" does not mean doubling your caloric intake. Instead, it's about nourishing your body and your baby with balanced, nutrient-rich foods. This chapter will discuss general nutritional guidelines for pregnancy and potential adjustments for traditional African or Caribbean diets to meet these guidelines.

General Nutrition Guidelines for Pregnancy

During pregnancy, the demand for certain nutrients, including protein, iron, calcium, folic acid, and specific vitamins, increases significantly.

1. **Protein:** A vital building block for your baby's cells, aim for 75 to 100 grams of protein per day. This can come from lean meats, poultry, fish, eggs, dairy, beans, and nuts.
2. **Iron:** Iron helps make hemoglobin for you and your baby. Sources include lean meats, beans, and iron-fortified cereals. Pair iron-rich foods with Vitamin C-rich foods to enhance absorption.
3. **Calcium:** Essential for your baby's bone development, aim for at least 1,000 milligrams per day. Dairy products, fortified plant milks, and leafy green vegetables are good sources.
4. **Folic Acid:** Crucial for preventing neural tube defects, aim for at least 600

micrograms per day. Sources include leafy green vegetables, fortified cereals, and legumes.

5. **Vitamins D and B12:** Vitamin D helps bone development, while B12 supports the formation of red blood cells and neurological function. Both are found in dairy products, eggs, and fortified foods.

Adjusting Traditional African and Caribbean Diets

Traditional African and Caribbean diets are often rich in starches, fiber, and fruits, while being low in fats. Here are a few suggestions to meet the increased nutritional needs of pregnancy:

1. **Increase Protein Intake:** Traditional African and Caribbean diets can be low in protein. Consider adding more lean meats, poultry, fish, or plant-based proteins like beans, lentils, and tofu to your meals.
2. **Ensure Adequate Iron and Folic Acid:** Include more leafy greens, legumes, and fortified cereals to increase your intake of these essential nutrients. Cooking in cast-iron pots can also increase iron content in your food.
3. **Add Healthy Fats:** Healthy fats are essential for your baby's brain development. Avocado, nuts, seeds, and fatty fish can be good additions to your diet.
4. **Limit Salt and Sugar:** Hypertension and gestational diabetes are common in Black women. Minimize added sugars and high-sodium foods in your diet.

Remember, everyone's nutritional needs and responses to pregnancy are unique. What works best will depend on your individual circumstances, including your pre-pregnancy weight, whether you're carrying multiples, and your activity level.

It's always advisable to consult with a healthcare provider or a dietitian who respects your cultural dietary practices and can provide personalized advice. Good nutrition is not about strict limitations, but balance, variety, and enjoyment—keeping both you and your baby healthy.

6

Chapter 6: Exercise and Mental Health

Maintaining a regular exercise routine and prioritizing mental health during pregnancy can have far-reaching benefits. Exercise can help manage weight gain, boost mood, improve sleep, and increase stamina for labor. Mental health is equally important, as emotional well-being directly impacts both mother and baby. This chapter delves into safe exercise options during pregnancy and strategies for maintaining mental health.

Exercise During Pregnancy

Staying active during pregnancy can greatly enhance your health and well-being. Here's how to do it safely:

1. **Check with Your Healthcare Provider:** Before starting any exercise routine, it's crucial to consult with your healthcare provider, especially if you have any medical conditions.

2. **Choose Safe Activities:** Low-impact activities like brisk walking, swimming, prenatal yoga, and stationary biking are generally safe for most pregnant women. Strength training can also be beneficial, but it's important to avoid heavy weights and exercises that involve lying flat on your back.

3. **Listen to Your Body:** Pregnancy is not the time to push your limits. If you feel any discomfort, pain, or other unusual symptoms, stop exercising

and contact your healthcare provider.

4. **Stay Hydrated and Cool:** Drink plenty of water before, during, and after exercising. Avoid overheating, particularly during the first trimester.

Mental Health During Pregnancy

Pregnancy can bring a mix of emotions, and it's normal to experience mood swings due to hormonal changes. However, serious and persistent feelings of sadness, anxiety, or emptiness should not be overlooked.

1. **Recognize the Signs:** Be aware of symptoms of depression and anxiety, which can include persistent sadness, extreme irritability, feelings of hopelessness, and excessive worrying.
2. **Seek Professional Help:** If you experience any signs of depression or anxiety, it's important to seek help promptly. Mental health professionals can provide treatments such as therapy, medication, or both.
3. **Build a Support Network:** Connecting with supportive family, friends, or support groups can provide emotional assistance.
4. **Practice Self-Care:** Engage in activities that you enjoy and relax you. This could be reading, meditation, prenatal yoga, or simply taking a warm bath.
5. **Stay Physically Active:** Regular physical activity can boost your mood and help manage anxiety and mild depression.
6. **Nutrition:** Eating a balanced diet can help maintain stable blood sugar levels, contributing to better mood regulation.

Pregnancy is a time of significant change, both physically and emotionally. By prioritizing your physical health through exercise and nurturing your mental well-being, you're taking critical steps toward a healthier pregnancy and a brighter start for your baby. If you ever feel overwhelmed, remember that it's okay to seek help—you don't have to navigate this journey alone.

7

Chapter 7: Identifying and Addressing Unique Risks

Black women face unique health risks during pregnancy that contribute to higher maternal mortality and morbidity rates. This chapter will critically analyze these risks and present strategies to mitigate them.

Unique Health Risks

Several factors contribute to the higher health risks experienced by Black pregnant women. Understanding these risks is the first step toward addressing them:

1. **Hypertensive Disorders:** Black women are more likely to experience hypertensive disorders, including preeclampsia, which can lead to severe complications such as stroke.
2. **Gestational Diabetes:** Black women have a higher risk of developing gestational diabetes, which can lead to complications such as premature birth and future type 2 diabetes.
3. **Preterm Birth:** Black women are more likely to give birth prematurely, which can cause health problems for the baby.
4. **Low Birth Weight:** Infants born to Black women are more likely to have low birth weight, putting them at higher risk for health problems.

5. **Maternal Mortality:** Due to a combination of systemic, social, and health factors, Black women are more likely to die from pregnancy-related causes.

Addressing These Risks

Addressing these unique risks involves personal care strategies, access to quality healthcare, and advocating for systemic changes:

1. **Prenatal Care:** Regular prenatal care can help identify and manage risks early.
2. **Healthy Lifestyle:** Regular exercise, a balanced diet, maintaining a healthy weight, and avoiding harmful substances can help manage risks like gestational diabetes and hypertensive disorders.
3. **Healthcare Provider Communication:** Establishing clear and open communication with your healthcare provider can help ensure your concerns are addressed.
4. **Self-Advocacy:** Advocate for yourself in the healthcare system. Don't hesitate to ask questions, seek second opinions, or express concerns.
5. **Support Network:** A strong support network of family, friends, and community organizations can provide emotional support, help you navigate the healthcare system, and advocate for your rights.
6. **Mental Health Care:** Access to mental health resources is crucial. Stress and depression can negatively impact both mother and baby and can contribute to preterm birth and low birth weight.
7. **Systemic Change:** Advocating for systemic changes in healthcare can address racial disparities in maternal health. This includes supporting policies that improve access to quality care for Black women and pushing for diversity and bias training in the medical field.

By identifying and understanding the unique risks Black pregnant women face, you're better equipped to take proactive steps to safeguard your health and the health of your baby. Remember, you're not alone in this journey—utilize your community, healthcare providers, and resources at your disposal to support a healthy pregnancy.

8

Chapter 8: Insurance: Your Safety Net

Health insurance can seem complex, but it's a crucial tool for navigating healthcare during your pregnancy. Understanding your coverage, rights, and how to effectively utilize your insurance benefits can help ensure you and your baby get the necessary care. This chapter provides a detailed guide to these aspects.

Understanding Maternity Coverage

Under the Affordable Care Act (ACA), all qualified health plans are required to cover maternity care, also referred to as "maternity and newborn care," one of the ten essential health benefits.

This coverage generally includes:

1. **Prenatal Care:** Regular check-ups, screenings, and lab tests.
2. **Inpatient Services:** Care received when you're admitted to a hospital, like labor and delivery services.
3. **Postnatal Care:** Follow-up visits after your baby's birth to check on your health and recovery.
4. **Breastfeeding Support:** Access to lactation counseling and breast pump rental coverage.

Understanding Your Rights

Understanding your rights can help you advocate for yourself and get the most from your insurance:

1. **Right to Maternity Care:** The ACA prohibits insurance companies from refusing to cover you or charging you more due to pre-existing conditions, including pregnancy.
2. **Right to Breastfeeding Support:** Insurers are required to cover breastfeeding support and equipment without cost-sharing.
3. **Right to Appeal Decisions:** If an insurance claim is denied, you have the right to appeal the decision and ask for an external review.
4. **Right to Special Enrollment Period:** The birth of a baby qualifies you for a Special Enrollment Period, allowing you to make changes to your health insurance.

Effectively Utilizing Your Insurance

Here are some steps to help you navigate and utilize your insurance benefits effectively:

1. **Review Your Policy:** Understand what your policy covers and what out-of-pocket costs (like co-pays and deductibles) you might be responsible for.
2. **Check Provider Network:** Confirm if your healthcare provider is in-network, as out-of-network providers can result in higher costs.
3. **Pre-Authorizations:** Some services may require pre-authorization from your insurance company. Check this in advance to avoid surprise bills.
4. **Document Everything:** Keep a record of all interactions with your insurance company and healthcare provider. This can be valuable if you need to dispute a bill or claim.
5. **Ask Questions:** If you don't understand something, ask. Whether it's your insurance company, doctor, or a hospital billing department, it's their job to help you understand.

Remember, it's okay to ask for help. Insurance can be complex, but resources are available. Patient advocates, social workers, and non-profit organizations can provide assistance. Understanding and effectively utilizing your insurance can ensure that you get the care you need for a healthy pregnancy.

9

Chapter 9: Advocacy and Self-Empowerment

As a Black woman navigating the healthcare system, self-advocacy is a powerful tool. By speaking up, asking questions, and demanding respectful and adequate care, you can greatly influence your pregnancy experience and outcomes. This chapter presents strategies for self-advocacy and empowerment.

Knowing Your Rights

Understanding your rights as a patient is the foundation of self-advocacy. You have the right to:

1. **Respectful and Non-Discriminatory Care:** You should be treated with dignity, respect, and without any discrimination.
2. **Informed Consent:** You have the right to be informed about all aspects of your care, and the right to accept or refuse treatment.
3. **Privacy and Confidentiality:** Your personal health information should be kept confidential and shared only with your consent.

Strategies for Advocacy and Self-Empowerment

Once you're aware of your rights, you can utilize the following strategies to ensure they're upheld:

1. **Speak Up and Ask Questions:** If something is unclear, ask for clarification. Your healthcare providers should be willing to answer your questions until you fully understand.
2. **Demand Respect:** If you feel disrespected, express your feelings directly and calmly. Ask for another healthcare provider if necessary.
3. **Know Your Care Plan:** Understanding your care plan helps you know what to expect and when to question if something feels off.
4. **Seek Second Opinions:** If you're unsure about a diagnosis or treatment plan, seeking a second opinion can provide reassurance or alternative options.
5. **Involve a Trusted Person:** Having a trusted person, such as a partner, family member, or doula, can provide support, offer a second set of ears, and help advocate for you during appointments or labor.
6. **Document Interactions:** Keeping a record of your interactions with healthcare providers can be useful, especially if a problem arises.
7. **Report Problems:** If you experience disrespectful care or discrimination, report it to the healthcare facility's patient advocate or administrator.

Community Resources and Advocacy Organizations

There are several organizations dedicated to improving the healthcare experience for Black women. These organizations provide resources, education, and platforms to share experiences:

1. **Black Mamas Matter Alliance:** An organization advocating for Black maternal health, rights, and justice.
2. **National Birth Equity Collaborative:** An organization working to reduce Black maternal and infant mortality through research, family services, and policy advocacy.
3. **SisterSong:** A reproductive justice collective for women of color.

By equipping yourself with knowledge, exercising your rights, and utilizing the support of your community, you can be a powerful advocate for your health and the health of your baby.

10

Chapter 10: Building Your Birth Plan

A birth plan is a document that communicates your preferences and expectations for labor and delivery to your healthcare team. While it's important to be flexible, as labor can be unpredictable, a birth plan provides a roadmap that respects your wishes and prepares for potential health scenarios. This chapter provides guidance on creating an effective birth plan.

Identifying Your Preferences

Start by considering your preferences for the following areas:

1. **Birth Setting:** Where do you feel most comfortable giving birth? This could be a hospital, a birth center, or at home.
2. **Labor Support:** Who do you want present during your labor and delivery? This could include a partner, family member, friend, or doula.
3. **Pain Management:** Consider your options for managing pain, such as epidurals, nitrous oxide, or natural methods like breathing exercises, birthing balls, and water birth.
4. **Labor Positions:** What positions do you prefer for labor and delivery?
5. **Fetal Monitoring:** How do you feel about continuous electronic fetal monitoring versus intermittent monitoring?
6. **Delivery Preferences:** Do you have any preferences for immediately after birth, such as delayed cord clamping or immediate skin-to-skin contact?

7. **Newborn Procedures:** What are your preferences for newborn procedures like vitamin K injection, eye ointment, and vaccinations?

Planning for Health Scenarios

Your birth plan should also account for potential health scenarios:

1. **Induction of Labor:** If your pregnancy goes past your due date or if complications arise, you might need to be induced. What are your thoughts on this?
2. **C-Section:** If a vaginal delivery isn't possible or safe, you may need a C-section. Include preferences for a family-centered (or "gentle") C-section, like immediate skin-to-skin contact, if possible.
3. **Preterm Birth:** If you go into labor prematurely, discuss preferences for the care of your baby, who may need to spend time in a neonatal intensive care unit (NICU).

Communicating Your Birth Plan

Once you've created your birth plan:

1. **Share with Your Healthcare Provider:** Discuss your birth plan with your healthcare provider. They can provide valuable feedback and help set realistic expectations.
2. **Share with Your Labor Support Team:** Make sure everyone who will be with you during labor and delivery understands your birth plan and can help advocate for your wishes.
3. **Be Flexible:** Understand that labor and delivery are unpredictable and you may need to deviate from your plan for the safety of you or your baby.

Creating a birth plan can give you a sense of control and peace of mind. Remember, the ultimate goal is a safe delivery and a healthy baby and mother. It's okay if things don't go exactly as planned; the important thing is that your wishes are considered and respected.

11

Chapter 11: Assembling Your Support System

A robust support system is instrumental in your pregnancy journey, providing emotional support, practical help, and advocacy when needed. This chapter will guide you on how to build and engage an effective support network.

Identifying Your Support Network

Your support network might include:

1. **Partner:** If applicable, your partner can provide emotional support, help with tasks, and serve as a key decision-maker.
2. **Family and Friends:** Loved ones can provide emotional support, practical help (like preparing meals, helping with housework or other children), and companionship.
3. **Doula:** A doula provides emotional, physical, and educational support during pregnancy, labor, and postpartum.
4. **Community Groups:** Local or online groups for expecting parents can offer peer support, advice, and friendship.
5. **Healthcare Team:** Your doctors, nurses, midwives, and other medical professionals are a critical part of your support network.

Engaging Your Support Network

Once you have identified your support network, here's how you can engage them:

1. **Communication:** Regularly communicate with your support network about your experiences, needs, and concerns. This will help them understand how they can best support you.
2. **Education:** Encourage your support network to learn about pregnancy, childbirth, and newborn care. This will equip them to provide informed support and advocacy.
3. **Emotional Support:** Be open about your feelings and emotions. Pregnancy can bring a range of emotions, and it's important for your support network to be aware and supportive.
4. **Practical Help:** Don't be afraid to ask for practical help, whether it's accompanying you to prenatal visits, helping with housework, or providing meals.
5. **Advocacy:** Ensure your support network knows your birth plan and is prepared to advocate for your preferences in the healthcare system.
6. **Postpartum Support:** Discuss your postpartum plan with your support network. Postpartum can be an emotionally and physically challenging time, and having your support system ready to help is critical.

A strong support network can provide emotional stability, practical help, and informed advocacy throughout your pregnancy journey. Remember, it's okay to ask for help. Pregnancy is a demanding time, and you don't have to navigate it alone. The people in your life want to be there for you—let them.

12

Chapter 12: Facing Discrimination: Your Rights and Recourses

While we aspire to an equitable healthcare system, the reality is that racial bias and discrimination still exist. As a Black pregnant woman, it's crucial to understand your rights and what to do if you experience discrimination. This chapter educates on these rights and outlines actionable steps for recourse.

Understanding Your Rights

As a patient, you have several rights:

1. **Respectful Care:** You have the right to receive care that is respectful, considerate, and free from discrimination.
2. **Informed Consent:** You have the right to receive all necessary information about your medical condition, treatment options, and risks, and you have the right to accept or refuse treatment.
3. **Privacy and Confidentiality:** You have the right to have your medical information kept private and shared only with your consent.
4. **Access to Medical Records:** You have the right to view and obtain copies of your medical records.
5. **Second Opinion:** You have the right to seek a second opinion if you're unsure about a diagnosis or treatment.

Addressing Discrimination

If you experience racial bias or discrimination, here are steps you can take:

1. **Speak Up:** If you're comfortable doing so, directly address the discriminatory behavior with the person involved, clearly stating that you believe their actions or comments are inappropriate and discriminatory.
2. **Report:** File a formal complaint with the healthcare provider, hospital or clinic's administration, or patient advocate.
3. **Document:** Keep a detailed record of each instance of discrimination, including dates, people involved, what was said or done, and any actions taken.
4. **Witnesses:** If there were any witnesses, include their accounts in your documentation.
5. **Legal Recourse:** If your complaints aren't addressed, consider seeking legal advice. Civil rights laws protect you from discrimination in healthcare settings.

Support Resources

Several organizations work to combat racial discrimination in healthcare:

1. **NAACP (National Association for the Advancement of Colored People):** Offers resources and support for individuals experiencing racial discrimination.
2. **Black Women's Health Imperative:** This organization advocates for Black women's health rights and provides resources to address healthcare discrimination.
3. **ACLU (American Civil Liberties Union):** Provides resources on healthcare rights and discrimination.

Experiencing racial bias or discrimination can be emotionally taxing. Don't hesitate to seek support from your network and mental health professionals. It's essential to prioritize your wellbeing, and there are people and organizations ready to stand with you in your fight for respectful, equitable care.

13

Chapter 13: Preparing for Maternity Leave

Preparing for maternity leave involves understanding your legal rights, negotiating with your employer, and planning financially to ensure a smooth transition. This chapter provides an overview of these steps and gives guidance on how to approach them.

Understanding Your Rights

In the United States, the Family and Medical Leave Act (FMLA) provides certain employees with up to 12 weeks of unpaid, job-protected leave per year, which can be used for the birth and care of a newborn. It also requires that their group health benefits be maintained during the leave.

To be eligible for FMLA leave, you must:

1. Work for a covered employer (generally private employers with 50 or more employees, public agencies, and public and private elementary and secondary schools)
2. Have worked for the employer for at least 12 months
3. Have worked at least 1,250 hours over the past 12 months
4. Work at a location where the employer has at least 50 employees within 75 miles

Negotiating Maternity Leave

If your employer does not offer paid maternity leave, or if you need more time than is offered, you may need to negotiate. Here's how:

1. **Research:** Understand the maternity leave policies of your employer and comparable companies in your industry.
2. **Plan:** Develop a proposal that outlines the length of your leave, how your work will be covered, and any flexibility you might have (e.g., working from home or part-time initially).
3. **Communicate:** Meet with your supervisor or human resources department to discuss your plan.

Financial Planning

Having a baby can significantly impact your financial situation, especially if your maternity leave is unpaid. Consider these steps:

1. **Budget:** Create a detailed budget to understand your income and expenses during your maternity leave.
2. **Save:** If possible, start saving money in advance of your maternity leave to help cover expenses during that time.
3. **Understand Your Benefits:** Look into any short-term disability insurance, accrued vacation or sick time, or other benefits you have that could help during this time.
4. **Government Assistance:** Investigate government assistance programs, such as the Women, Infants, and Children (WIC) program, which can help with the costs of food and baby supplies.

Preparation is key when it comes to maternity leave. By understanding your rights, effectively negotiating with your employer, and financially planning, you can ensure your transition into motherhood is as smooth as possible.

14

Chapter 14: The Home Stretch: Third Trimester

As you enter the third trimester, you are on the final stretch of your pregnancy. This period, often from week 28 until birth, is filled with excitement, anticipation, and a myriad of physical changes. This chapter discusses common discomforts of the third trimester and preparations for birth.

Understanding the Third Trimester

During the third trimester, your baby grows rapidly, and you might notice changes such as:

1. **Weight Gain:** You'll likely gain several pounds as your baby grows.
2. **Increased Discomfort:** As your baby grows, you may experience back pain, difficulty sleeping, shortness of breath, heartburn, and swelling in your ankles, fingers, and face.
3. **Breasts:** Your breasts may become larger and leak small amounts of fluid, a precursor to breast milk called colostrum.
4. **Frequent Urination:** The increased pressure on your bladder from your growing uterus may cause you to urinate more frequently.
5. **Braxton Hicks Contractions:** Often called "practice contractions," Braxton Hicks contractions can be felt as a tightening in your abdomen

but are typically irregular and do not open your cervix.

Preparations for Birth

1. **Understand the Signs of Labor:** These may include regular contractions, water breaking, or a pink or brownish discharge known as "bloody show."
2. **Complete Your Nursery:** Ensure your baby's sleeping area is ready and safe.
3. **Pack a Hospital Bag:** Include essentials for you and the baby, such as clothes, toiletries, a car seat, and your birth plan.
4. **Take a Childbirth Class:** Such classes can help you feel more prepared for labor and delivery.
5. **Decide on Pain Management:** Talk to your healthcare provider about your options for managing labor pain.
6. **Plan for Postpartum:** Organize your home and support system to make the transition easier after the baby arrives.

The third trimester is a time of physical discomfort, but also immense excitement. Take time to rest, prepare, and anticipate the arrival of your new baby. Remember, it's okay to ask for help, and regular communication with your healthcare provider can help you navigate this period with more ease and confidence.

15

Chapter 15: Birth Settings: Making Informed Choices

C hoosing where to give birth is a crucial decision. The birth setting impacts the experience, interventions, and healthcare providers available to you during labor and delivery. This chapter explores the advantages and considerations of various birth settings and guides you in making an informed decision.

Hospital Births

Most American women give birth in hospitals, which offer a range of medical resources and emergency care if needed.

Advantages:

1. Access to medical professionals and technology for high-risk pregnancies.
2. Immediate access to a cesarean section or other interventions if necessary.
3. Anesthesiologists available for pain management options like epidurals.

Considerations:

1. Hospitals often have more rigid protocols, which might limit movement

or choice of birthing positions.

2. The environment can feel impersonal or clinical.
3. Higher rates of medical interventions, such as inductions and C-sections.

Birth Center Births

Birth centers are a homelike environment where care is provided by midwives. They are typically designed for low-risk pregnancies.

Advantages:

1. More personal and homelike environment.
2. Greater freedom to move around and choose birthing positions.
3. Lower rates of medical intervention.

Considerations:

1. If complications arise, transfer to a hospital may be necessary.
2. Pain relief options may be limited.
3. Not all insurance companies cover birth center care.

Home Births

Home births offer the opportunity to labor and deliver in the comfort of your own home, typically with a midwife.

Advantages:

1. Familiar, comfortable environment.
2. Significant control over your labor and delivery process.
3. Lower rates of medical intervention.

Considerations:

1. In the event of a complication, hospital transfer is necessary, which could delay emergency care.
2. Not all midwives have the same level of training or experience.

3. Not all insurance companies cover home births.

Making the Choice

When deciding, consider:

1. **Your Health and Risk Factors:** Certain conditions might make one setting more suitable than another.
2. **Your Personal Preferences:** Consider your desires for the birthing experience, including the atmosphere and available interventions.
3. **Access and Insurance:** Your options may be influenced by what is available in your area and what your insurance will cover.
4. **Healthcare Provider's Opinion:** Discuss the options with your healthcare provider. They can provide insight based on your specific health circumstances.

Remember, there is no universally right or wrong choice – only the choice that feels right for you and your baby, considering all factors. Be sure to explore each option thoroughly, ask questions, and make an informed decision that aligns with your health, comfort, and personal preferences.

16

Chapter 16: The Birth Process and Emergency Preparedness

Understanding the birth process and preparing for potential emergencies is crucial to ensure the safest possible outcome for both mother and baby. This chapter provides an in-depth view of what to expect during labor and delivery and outlines how to prepare for unexpected situations.

Understanding the Birth Process

The birth process typically involves three stages:

1. **First Stage (Dilation):** This stage starts with the onset of labor and ends when the cervix is fully dilated at 10 centimeters. It's typically the longest stage and can be further divided into early, active, and transitional phases.

2. **Second Stage (Pushing and Birth):** This stage starts once the cervix is fully dilated and ends with the birth of the baby. The mother will feel an urge to push during contractions, working with her body and healthcare provider to birth the baby.

3. **Third Stage (Delivery of the Placenta):** After the baby is born, contractions will continue until the placenta is delivered. This stage usually takes 5 to 30 minutes.

Potential Complications and Emergencies

While many births proceed without significant complications, it's important to be aware of potential issues:

1. **Prolonged Labor:** Also known as failure to progress, this occurs when labor lasts for about 20 hours or more for first-time mothers, and 14 hours or more for those who have given birth before.
2. **Perineal Tears:** These are common during childbirth, especially for first-time mothers. Severe tears can lead to long-term complications.
3. **Postpartum Hemorrhage:** This is excessive bleeding following childbirth and can be life-threatening if not managed promptly.
4. **Preterm Labor:** This is labor that begins too early, before 37 weeks of pregnancy.
5. **Umbilical Cord Issues:** These can include the cord being wrapped around the baby's neck or a prolapsed cord, which is when the cord comes out of the uterus before the baby.
6. **Placental Abruption:** This is a serious condition in which the placenta detaches from the uterus before the baby is born.
7. **Preeclampsia:** This is a pregnancy complication characterized by high blood pressure and signs of damage to other organ systems.

Emergency Preparedness

While it's impossible to predict every potential complication, having a plan can help ensure you get the necessary care quickly:

1. **Know the Signs:** Be aware of the signs of common complications and don't hesitate to contact your healthcare provider if you notice anything unusual.
2. **Have a Plan:** Talk to your healthcare provider about what to do and where to go if you experience complications during labor or after birth.
3. **Stay Flexible:** Understand that birth plans might need to be altered for the safety of you and your baby.
4. **Know Your Healthcare Team:** Ensure you have reliable contacts in your

healthcare team, and don't hesitate to ask questions or voice concerns.

5. **Postpartum Checkups:** Attend all postpartum checkups to monitor your recovery and catch any potential issues early.

Remember, while it's important to be informed and prepared, try not to let the fear of complications overshadow the joy of your pregnancy and birth. Trust in your healthcare team, and don't hesitate to reach out to them with any concerns or questions.

17

Chapter 17: Postpartum Care and Recovery

The postpartum period, also known as the "fourth trimester," is a time of physical recovery and emotional adjustment. This chapter provides guidance on postpartum self-care, newborn care, breastfeeding, and navigating the changes that come during this period.

Physical Recovery

Recovering from childbirth is a gradual process and varies for each woman. Here's what you might expect:

1. **Bleeding:** After birth, you'll experience lochia, a discharge made of blood and tissue from your uterus. This can last for several weeks and should gradually lighten.

2. **Pain and Healing:** If you had a vaginal birth, you might experience soreness, perineal discomfort, or hemorrhoids. For C-sections, you'll be healing from abdominal surgery. Over-the-counter medications or prescribed pain relief can help, as can techniques like warm baths or ice packs.

3. **Breast Changes:** Whether or not you're breastfeeding, your breasts will likely become engorged as they start producing milk. Breastfeeding or pumping can alleviate the pressure, while ice packs or chilled cabbage leaves can offer relief if you're not breastfeeding.

Newborn Care

Caring for your newborn might feel overwhelming at first, but you'll quickly learn to understand your baby's needs. Key areas include:

1. **Feeding:** Breast milk or formula will be your baby's primary source of nutrition. Newborns typically need to feed every 2-3 hours, or 8-12 times a day.
2. **Diapering:** You'll be changing many diapers each day. Be sure to clean the area gently but thoroughly and look out for signs of diaper rash.
3. **Sleeping:** Newborns sleep a lot but in short bursts. Safe sleep guidelines recommend placing your baby on their back in a crib with a firm mattress.

Breastfeeding

Breastfeeding is a learning process for both you and your baby. Key aspects include:

1. **Latch:** A good latch is essential for effective feeding and preventing sore nipples. Seek help from a lactation consultant if you have difficulties.
2. **Feeding on Demand:** Feed your baby whenever they show signs of hunger, such as sucking motions, reaching for the breast, or becoming more alert.
3. **Support:** If you're struggling with breastfeeding, reach out to lactation consultants, your healthcare provider, or breastfeeding support groups.

Adjusting to the Postpartum Period

The postpartum period is a time of adjustment. You might feel a range of emotions, from joy and amazement to anxiety or sadness.

1. **Emotional Health:** It's normal to have some degree of "baby blues," but if feelings of sadness or anxiety persist, speak to your healthcare provider about postpartum depression.
2. **Rest:** Sleep when your baby sleeps and accept help from others to ensure you're getting the rest you need.
3. **Support Network:** Don't hesitate to lean on your support network,

whether that's your partner, family, friends, or a new parent support group.

4. **Self-Care:** Ensure you're eating a balanced diet, drinking plenty of fluids, and getting some gentle exercise.

The postpartum period is a transformative time. It's essential to remember to take care of yourself while adjusting to life with your new baby. Don't hesitate to seek help and support when you need it. You're not alone in this journey.

18

Chapter 18: Mental Health Postpartum

Mental health postpartum is just as important as physical health. This period is a time of major adjustment and hormonal changes, which can impact your emotions significantly. This chapter delves into the understanding and management of postpartum depression and anxiety, providing resources for help if needed.

Understanding Postpartum Depression and Anxiety

1. **Postpartum Depression (PPD):** PPD is a serious mental health condition that can occur in the weeks or months following childbirth. It's characterized by feelings of extreme sadness, hopelessness, low energy, and a lack of interest in things you once enjoyed. It can also impact your ability to care for your baby or yourself.
2. **Postpartum Anxiety (PPA):** PPA can manifest as intense worry, restlessness, and a fear of being alone with the baby. Women with PPA may also have physical symptoms, such as dizziness, hot flashes, and nausea.

Risk Factors

Factors that might increase the risk of developing PPD or PPA include:

1. A history of depression or anxiety, either during pregnancy or at other times.

2. Family history of mental health disorders.
3. A traumatic childbirth experience.
4. Lack of strong emotional support.
5. Being a first-time mother.

Getting Help

If you're experiencing symptoms of PPD or PPA, it's crucial to seek help. Remember, these conditions are not your fault, and you're not alone. Steps to take include:

1. **Speak Up:** Talk to your healthcare provider about what you're experiencing. They can refer you to mental health professionals who specialize in postpartum mental health.
2. **Therapy:** Cognitive-behavioral therapy (CBT) and interpersonal therapy (IPT) have been shown to be effective in treating PPD.
3. **Medication:** Antidepressants can be an effective treatment method for PPD or PPA. If you're breastfeeding, discuss with your healthcare provider as some medications are safe to use while breastfeeding.
4. **Support Groups:** Speaking with other mothers who are experiencing the same struggles can provide comfort, reduce feelings of isolation, and provide practical insight.

Self-Care Strategies

In addition to professional treatment, self-care strategies can help manage symptoms:

1. **Rest:** Sleep deprivation can exacerbate symptoms of depression and anxiety. Try to sleep when your baby sleeps and accept help from others to allow you to rest.
2. **Healthy Eating:** Maintain a diet rich in fruits, vegetables, lean protein, and whole grains. Certain nutrients, like omega-3 fatty acids, have been linked to improved mood.
3. **Exercise:** Physical activity can boost your mood by increasing the

production of endorphins, your body's natural 'feel-good' chemicals.

4. **Mindfulness and Relaxation Techniques:** Practices like meditation, deep breathing, and yoga can help reduce symptoms of depression and anxiety.
5. **Stay Connected:** Stay in touch with family and friends, or join a local mothers' group. Talking to others about your experiences and feelings can be therapeutic.

Remember, taking care of your mental health is essential for both you and your baby. Don't hesitate to ask for help if you're feeling down or anxious. With the right help and treatment, you can fully recover from PPD or PPA and enjoy your time with your newborn.

19

Chapter 19: Ensuring Your Infant's Health

Ensuring your baby's health goes beyond basic care. You need to be aware of essential screenings, keep up with vaccinations, and choose a pediatrician who understands and respects your cultural background. This chapter aims to guide you through these crucial steps.

Newborn Screenings

Newborn screenings are tests that help identify conditions that might affect your baby's long-term health or survival. Early detection, diagnosis, and intervention can prevent death or disability and enable children to reach their full potential.

1. **Hearing Screening:** Most babies have a hearing test in the first few days after birth, ideally before leaving the hospital. Early identification of hearing loss will enable your child to get the support they need right from the start.

2. **Heart Defect Screening:** Using a simple, painless test called pulse oximetry, healthcare providers check for critical congenital heart defects (CCHDs).

3. **Metabolic/Genetic Screening:** A blood test typically checks for several inherited disorders. Early detection can allow for treatments that may prevent or lessen symptoms associated with the condition.

Vaccinations

Vaccinations are a critical part of preventing disease. They protect your child from serious illnesses and complications of vaccine-preventable diseases.

1. **Hepatitis B Vaccine:** The first dose is given soon after birth, usually within the first 24 hours.
2. **DTaP, Polio, Hib, Hepatitis B, Pneumococcal, and Rotavirus Vaccines:** These vaccinations are given over a series of visits, starting from 2 months of age.
3. **Flu Vaccine:** It's recommended yearly beginning at 6 months.

Choosing a Pediatrician

Choosing the right pediatrician for your child is an important decision. You'll want a doctor who is highly skilled, but also one who respects your cultural practices and understands your perspective.

1. **Credentials and Experience:** The pediatrician you choose should be certified by the Board of Pediatrics and have ample experience.
2. **Office Hours and Availability:** Consider the pediatrician's office hours. Ensure they align with your schedule and that there's a plan for handling emergencies or questions after hours.
3. **Communication Style:** The pediatrician should be someone you feel comfortable talking with and who takes the time to answer your questions.
4. **Cultural Competency:** This is the ability to interact effectively with people of different cultures. Your pediatrician should show respect for your beliefs and customs, and incorporate your cultural practices into your child's care when safe and possible.
5. **Healthcare Philosophy:** Ensure the pediatrician's approach to healthcare aligns with your own, especially concerning issues like breastfeeding, sleep training, and medication use.

Remember, as a parent, you are your child's best advocate. Trust your instincts, ask questions, and seek out the best care for your little one. Your active role can make a difference in ensuring your baby's health and wellbeing.

48

20

Chapter 20: Balancing Motherhood, Work, and Self-Care

Transitioning back to work while juggling new motherhood and maintaining self-care can be overwhelming. It requires careful planning, support, and a lot of patience with yourself. This chapter provides advice on how to balance these responsibilities and emphasizes the importance of continuous engagement with healthcare as a Black mother.

Transitioning Back to Work

1. **Plan Ahead:** Before your maternity leave ends, consider what your ideal work scenario would look like. Would you prefer a gradual return, part-time hours, or flexible scheduling? Talk to your employer to see what can be arranged.

2. **Practice Your New Routine:** A few days before returning to work, practice your new morning routine. This will give you a chance to work out any kinks before you actually have to be at work.

3. **Expect Emotions:** It's completely normal to have mixed feelings about going back to work. Remember, it's a significant transition, and it will take time to adjust.

Finding Quality Childcare

1. **Start Early:** Quality childcare often has a waiting list. Starting your search early will give you the best chance of securing a spot in your preferred program.
2. **Ask the Right Questions:** Inquire about caregiver qualifications, child-to-caregiver ratios, turn-over rates, and how they handle emergencies.
3. **Trust Your Instincts:** When you visit potential childcare providers, pay attention to how you feel. Do the children seem happy and engaged? Is the environment clean and safe?

Maintaining a Balance of Self-Care and Motherhood

1. **Schedule Self-Care:** Make time for activities you enjoy. This could be as simple as reading a book, going for a walk, or having a coffee with a friend.
2. **Stay Active:** Regular exercise can boost your mood, give you more energy, and help you sleep better. Even a short walk with your baby in the stroller can have significant benefits.
3. **Stay Connected:** Stay in touch with your friends, family, or join a mothers' group. Sharing experiences can help reduce feelings of isolation and provide emotional support.
4. **Ask for Help:** If you're feeling overwhelmed, don't hesitate to ask for help. Whether it's from your partner, a family member, a friend, or a professional, there's no shame in needing support.

Continuous Engagement with Healthcare as a Black Mother

1. **Regular Check-ups:** Ensure you have regular check-ups with your healthcare provider to monitor your physical and mental health.
2. **Be an Advocate:** Continue to advocate for yourself in healthcare settings. Don't be afraid to ask questions or seek a second opinion if something doesn't feel right.
3. **Health Education:** Stay informed about health issues that disproportionately affect Black women, such as hypertension and diabetes.

Remember, finding a balance between work, motherhood, and self-care doesn't mean doing everything perfectly. It's about making the best decisions for your mental, emotional, and physical health. It's about understanding your limits, asking for help when you need it, and taking one day at a time. It's your journey, and you're doing a great job.